Fit and Fabulous at 50" Unlock the Secrets to Looking 20 Again

"The Essential Blueprint for Effortless Weight Loss and Regaining Your Youthful Figure at 50+"

Maryqueen J.Toiu

Copyright © 2023 MaryqueenJ.Toiu

Table of Content

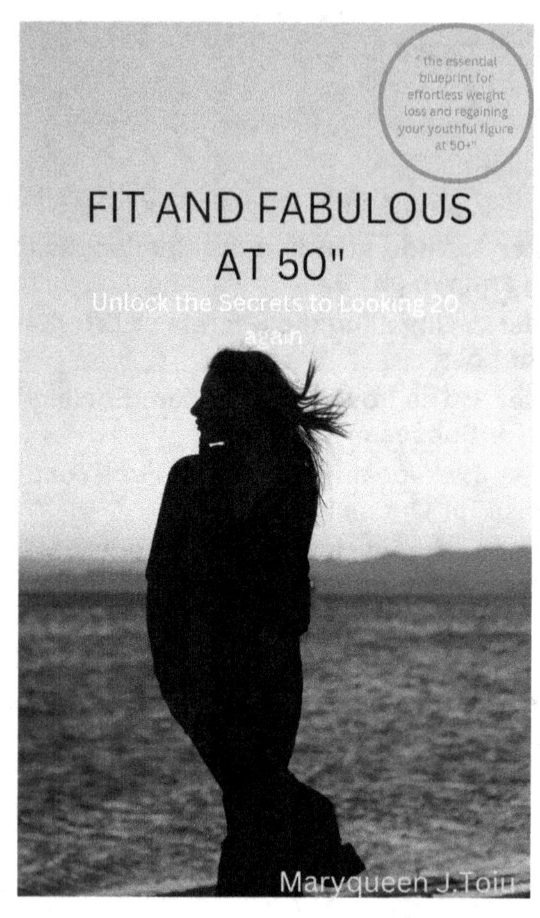
" the essential
blueprint for
effortless weight
loss and regaining
your youthful figure
at 50+"
FIT AND FABULOUS
AT 50"
Unlock the Secrets to Looking 20
again
Maryqueen J.Toiu

Introduction

Rediscovering Your Youthful Figure at 50+

Picture this: It's your 50th birthday, and you find yourself standing at the precipice of a new chapter in life. As you reflect on the years gone by, a glimmer of nostalgia for your youthful figure and vitality starts to flicker within you. You yearn to recapture that radiant energy, that sense of invincibility, and the confidence that came effortlessly in your twenties. You wonder if it's possible to turn back the clock and reclaim your youthful figure at 50 and beyond.

I'm here to assure you that it really is. Welcome to "Fit and Fabulous at 50: Unlock the Secrets to Looking 20 Again" – a groundbreaking guide that will empower you to rewrite the narrative of aging and rediscover the youthful figure you've always dreamt of. This isn't a quick fix; it's a transformative blueprint meticulously crafted to help you effortlessly shed those extra pounds, regain your energy, and radiate a youthful glow.

But how can this be possible, you may ask? Let me share a story with you. Meet Sarah, a remarkable woman who, like many of us, found herself doubting the possibility of reclaiming her youthful figure as she entered her fifties. Determined to prove that age isjust a number, Sarah embarked on a journey of self-discovery, armed with the tools and knowledge to unlock the secrets of looking 20 again.

Through Sarah's inspiring story and the expert guidance provided in this book, you will unlock the essential blueprint for effortless weight loss and regaining your youthful figure. You will delve into the science-backed strategies, discover the power of nutrition and exercise tailored specifically for your needs, and uncover the secrets of cultivating a positive mindset and self-care routine that will make you feel unstoppable.

But this is more than just a physical transformation; it's a journey of self-empowerment and self-acceptance. It's about embracing your age with grace and confidence, celebrating the wisdom and experience that come with it, while also nurturing your body and soul to look and feel your best.

Whether you've been searching for ways to shed those stubborn pounds, tone your muscles, or regain your energy and vitality, "Fit and Fabulous at 50" is the ultimate guide to help you unlock your full potential and rewrite the rules of aging.

So, if you're ready to embark on a remarkable journey of self-discovery, reclaim your youthful figure, and unlock the secrets to looking 20 again, get ready to dive into the pages of thisempowering and transformative book. It's time to embrace the possibilities that await you, defy societal norms, and uncover the true essence of your beauty, strength, and radiance. Welcome to "Fit and Fabulous at 50: Unlock the Secrets to Looking 20 Again" – your gateway to rediscovering your youthful figure at 50 and beyond. Let the journey begin.

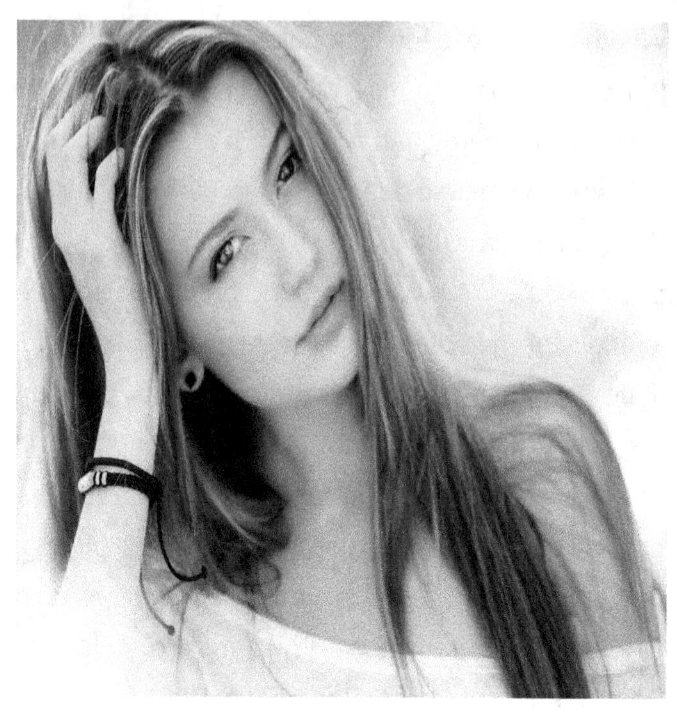

Chapter 1: Understanding the Challenges of Aging and Weight Gain

Aging and weight gain are two common challenges that many individuals face as they get older.
This chapter aims to provide an understanding of these challenges and explore their relationship.

The Aging Process:

A natural process that impacts all living things is aging.

As we age, our bodies undergo physiological changes, including a decrease in muscle mass, bone density, and metabolism.

These changes can result in weight gain and an increased risk of chronic diseases like diabetes and heart disease.

Factors Contributing to Weight Gain in Aging:

Several factors contribute to weight gain in aging, including hormonal changes, decreased physical activity, and changes in appetite and metabolism.

Hormonal changes, such as a decrease in estrogen levels in women during menopause, can lead to weight gain, particularly in the abdominal area.

Decreased physical activity, often due to decreased muscle mass, can result in a slower metabolism and weight gain.

Impact of Weight Gain on Aging:

Weight gain in aging can have significant implications for overall health and well-being.

Excess weight can increase the risk of developing chronic diseases, such as diabetes, heart disease, and certain types of cancer.

Weightgain can also lead to reduced mobility, increased joint pain, and diminished quality of life.

Strategies for Managing Weight Gain in Aging:

Despite the challenges, it is possible to manage weight gain in aging through various strategies.

Regular physical activity, including both cardiovascular and strength-training exercises, can help maintain muscle mass and boost metabolism.

Following a balanced and nutritious diet, rich in fruits, vegetables, lean proteins, and whole grains, can support healthy weight management.

- Adequate sleep, stress management, and staying hydrated are also important factors in maintaining a healthy weight.

Importance of Seeking Professional Guidance:

It is advisable to consult with a healthcare professional or a registered dietitian to develop a personalized plan for managing weight gain in aging.

They can assess individual needs, provide guidance on exercise and nutrition, and monitor progress.

Seeking professional guidance can ensure safe and effective weight management for older individuals.

Understanding the challenges of aging and weight gain is crucial for promoting healthy aging.

By adopting lifestyle changes, seeking professional guidance, and prioritizing self-care, individuals can effectively manage weight gain and improve overall well-being as they age.

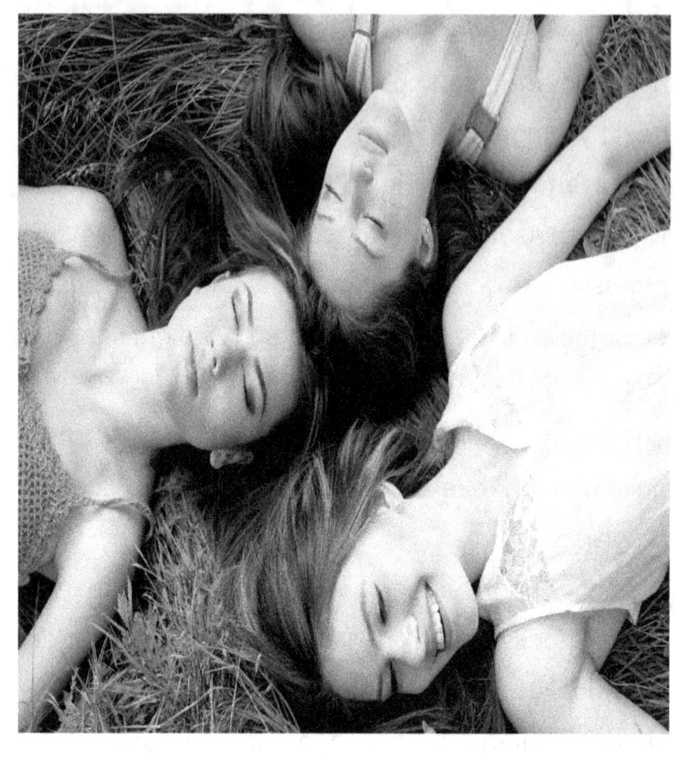

Chapter 2: Unveiling the Secrets to Effortless Weight Loss

A typical objective for many people looking to enhance their general health and well-being is weight loss.

This chapter aims to uncover the secrets to achieving effortless weight loss by understanding the factors that contribute to weight gain and implementing effective strategies for sustainable weight loss.

Factors Contributing to Weight Gain:

Before diving into weight loss techniques, it is essential to understand the factors that contribute to weight gain.

These factors include an unhealthy diet, lack of physical activity, hormonal imbalances, emotional eating, and lifestyle habits.

By addressing these factors, individuals can lay the foundation for successful and sustainable weight loss.

Mindset Shift:

A crucial step towards effortless weight loss is cultivating a positive and motivated mindset.

Adopting a growth mindset and believing in one's ability to change and achieve weight loss goals is vital.

It is important to focus on progress rather than perfection and to embrace self-compassion throughout the weight loss journey.

Establishing Healthy Eating Habits:

Implementing healthy eating habits is essential for sustainable weight loss.

This includes consuming a well-balanced diet rich in fruits, vegetables, whole grains, lean proteins, andhealthy fats.

Portion control, mindful eating, and listening to the body's hunger and fullness cues are important practices to adopt.

Avoiding crash diets or restrictive eating patterns is crucial, as they often lead to weight regain and unhealthy relationships with food.

Regular Physical Activity:

Incorporating regular physical activity into daily routines is key for effortless weight loss.

Engaging in both cardiovascular exercises and strength training helps burn calories, build lean muscle mass, and boost metabolism.

Finding activities that are enjoyable and sustainable, such as walking, dancing, or cycling, increases the likelihood of sticking to an exercise routine.

Stress Management:

Chronic stress can contribute to weight gain and hinder weight loss efforts.

Learning effective stress management techniques, such as meditation, deep breathing exercises, and engaging in hobbies, can help mitigate the negative impact of stress on weight loss.

Prioritizing self-care and finding healthy ways to cope with stress are essential components of achieving effortless weight loss.

Support and Accountability:

Seeking support and accountability from loved ones or joining a weight loss program or support group can greatly enhance weight loss success.

Having a support system provides encouragement, motivation, and a sense of community, which can be crucial during challenging moments.

Regularcheck-ins and progress tracking with a trusted friend or a healthcare professional can help individuals stay accountable and make necessary adjustments to their weight loss plan.

Sustainable Lifestyle Changes:

Effortless weight loss is not about quick fixes or temporary solutions. It is about making sustainable lifestyle changes.

Gradual, small changes that can be maintained long-term are more effective than drastic measures. Setting realistic goals and focusing on long-term health and well-being, rather than just a number on the scale, ensures sustainable and lasting weight loss.

Celebrating Non-Scale Victories:

Effortless weight loss is not solely determined by the number on the scale.

Celebrating non-scale victories, such as increased energy, improved sleep, enhanced mood, or fitting into smaller clothes, helps foster a positive mindset and overall well-being.

These non-scale victories serve as powerful motivators and reminders of the progress being made.

Effortless weight loss is within reach for individuals who are committed to making sustainable lifestyle changes.

By understanding the factors contributing to weight gain, adopting a positive mindset, establishing healthy eating habits, engaging in regular physical activity, managing stress, seeking support, and celebrating non-scale victories, individuals can achieve their weight loss goals and maintaina healthy weight effortlessly. The journey towards effortless weight loss is not always easy, but with perseverance, determination, and a focus on long-term health and well-being, it is attainable.

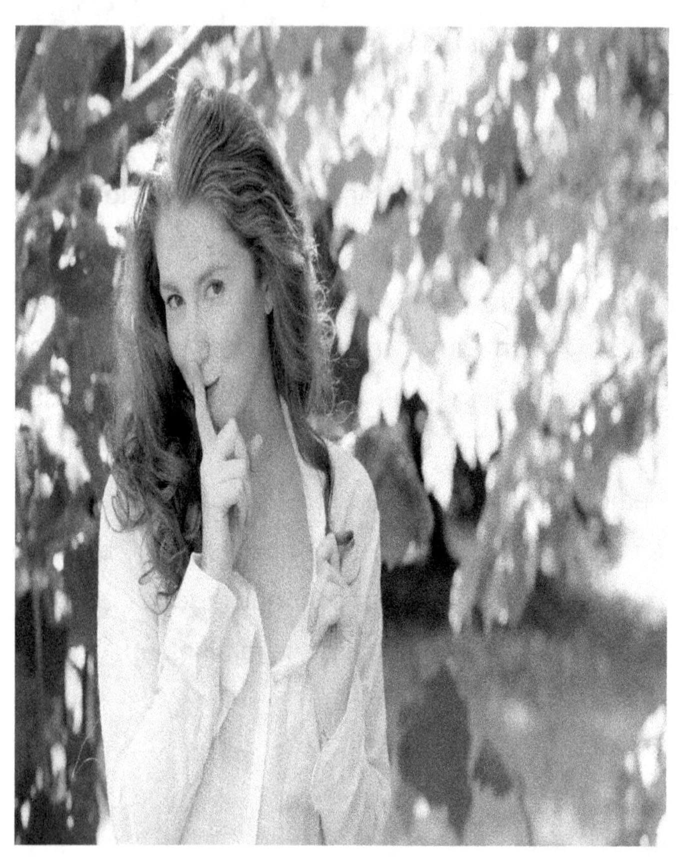

Chapter 3: The Power of Nutrition: Fueling Your Body for Success

In order to achieve success, it is crucial to fuel your body with the right nutrition. The food we consume plays a vital role in our overall health and well-being. It provides us with the energy and nutrients needed to perform at our best and achieve our goals. In this chapter, we will explore the power of nutrition and how it can fuel your body for success.

One of the first things to understand about nutrition is that it goes beyond simply counting calories. It is about nourishing your body with the right balance of macronutrients – carbohydrates, proteins, and fats – as well as micronutrients like vitamins and minerals. Each of these nutrients has a specific role to play in our bodies, and it is important to consume the right amount of each to support optimal function.

Carbohydrates are the body's main source of energy. They provide fuel for the brain and muscles, enabling us to think clearly and perform physical tasks. However, not all carbohydrates are created equal. It is important to choose complex carbohydrates, such as whole grains, fruits, and vegetables, as they provide a slow and steady release of energy, keeping us energized throughout the day. Simple carbohydrates, on the other hand, like processed sugars, can lead to energy crashes and cravings.

Building and mending tissues as well as boosting the immune system depend on proteins.They are made up of amino acids, which are the building blocks of protein. It is important to consume a variety of protein sources, such as lean meats, fish, eggs, dairy products, legumes, and nuts, to ensure you are getting all the essential amino acids your body needs.

Fats often get a bad reputation, but they are an important part of a healthy diet. Healthy fats, like those found in avocados, nuts, seeds, and olive oil, are beneficial for brain health, reducing inflammation, and supporting hormone production. It is important to limit unhealthy fats, like trans fats and saturated fats, found in processed foods and fried foods, as they can increase the risk of heart disease and other health problems.

In addition to macronutrients, it is important to consume a wide variety of micronutrients. These include vitamins, such as vitamin C, vitamin D, and vitamin E, as well as minerals like calcium, iron, and magnesium. Numerous biological processes, such as immune system support, bone health, and energy production, depend on these nutrients.

Fueling your body with the right nutrition not only supports physical health but also mental and emotional well-being. Studieshave shown that a healthy diet can improve mood, reduce stress, and enhance cognitive function. Eating a balanced diet that includes a variety of fruits, vegetables, whole grains, lean proteins, and healthy fats can help stabilize blood sugar levels, promote proper digestion, and provide the necessary nutrients for optimal brain function.

In order to fuel your body for success, it is important to pay attention to portion sizes and listen to your body's hunger and fullness cues. It is not just about what you eat, but also how much you eat. Overeating can lead to weight gain, sluggishness, and decreased energy levels, while under-eating can leave you feeling weak and depleted.

Meal planning and preparation can also play a key role in fueling your body for success. By planning your meals and snacks ahead of time, you can ensure that you have nutritious options readily available, even when life gets busy. This can help prevent impulsive food choices, like grabbing unhealthy fast food, and allow you to make more mindful decisions about what you put into your body.

Lastly, hydration is another essential component of proper nutrition. Drinking enough water throughout the day is essential for maintaining overall health and ensuring optimal bodily functions. Water helps to transport nutrients, regulate body temperature, and remove waste products from thebody. Dehydration can lead to fatigue, headaches, and decreased cognitive function, so it is important to drink water regularly and stay hydrated.

In conclusion, nutrition is a powerful tool for fueling your body for success. By providing your body with the right balance of macronutrients and micronutrients, you can support optimal physical and mental health. Proper nutrition can provide the energy and nutrients needed to perform at your best, maintain focus and concentration, and support overall well-being. By making mindful choices about what you put into your body and taking care of your nutrition, you can set yourself up for success in all areas of your life.

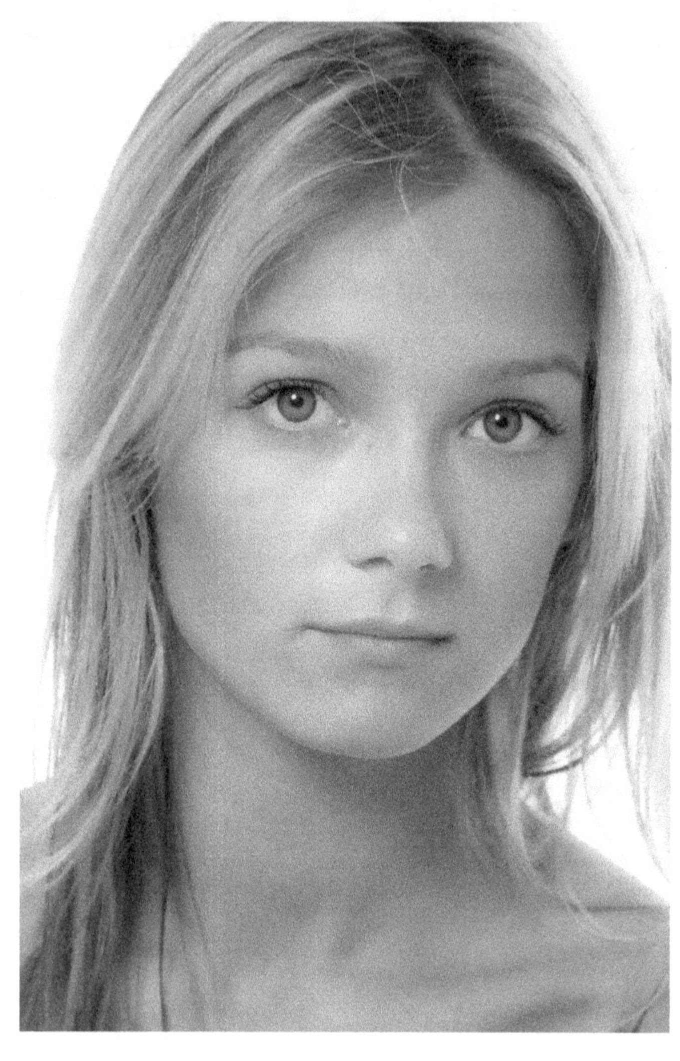

Chapter 4: Unlocking the Fountain of Youth: Exercise for Optimal Health

Exercise is not just beneficial for weight loss or to improve physical appearance. Regular exercise is vital for optimal health and can have numerous positive effects on our bodies and minds. In this chapter, we will explore the importance of exercise for maintaining youthfulness and overall well-being.

Introduction to Exercise for Optimal Health:

Regular physical activity is crucial for maintaining good health at any age. Exercise helps to strengthen our muscles, maintain a healthy weight, boost energy levels, improve cardiovascular health, and reduce the risk of chronic diseases such as diabetes and heart disease. Along with these physical benefits, exercise also plays a significant role in supporting mental health, improving mood, alleviating stress, and promoting a sense of well-being.

The Connection Between Exercise and Youthfulness:

Exercise has been proven to have anti-aging effects on the body. It helps to improve muscle tone, flexibility, and overall physical strength, making individuals feel and look younger. Additionally, regular exercise helps to maintain healthy skin by improving blood circulation and promoting the delivery of essential nutrients to the skin cells, giving a youthful radiance to the skin.

Exercise and Longevity:

Studies have shown that regular exercise can increase lifespan and promotelongevity. Engaging in physical activity can reduce the risk of age-related diseases and conditions such as cardiovascular disease, osteoporosis, and cognitive decline. Exercise also helps to improve immune function, reduce inflammation, and enhance overall quality of life, allowing individuals to live longer and healthier lives.

Types of Exercises for Optimal Health:

There are various types of exercises that can help to achieve optimal health. Aerobic exercises such as walking, jogging, swimming, or cycling help to improve cardiovascular fitness and endurance. Strength training exercises, such as weightlifting or resistance training, help to build and maintain muscle strength. Flexibility exercises, such as yoga or Pilates, promote flexibility, balance, and improve posture. It is important to incorporate a combination of aerobic, strength, and flexibility exercises into your fitness routine for maximum benefits.

Guidelines for Exercising Safely:

While exercise is beneficial, it is important to exercise safely to avoid injury. It is recommended to consult with a healthcare professional or a certified fitness trainer before starting a new exercise program. Begin with low-impact workouts and progressively boost the time and intensity. Maintain proper form and technique during exercises and listen to your body. Do not push yourself too hard and always warm up and cool down before and after exercise sessions. Stay hydrated, wear appropriate workout attire and footwear, and pay attention to any signs of discomfort or pain. If you have any underlying health conditions or injuries, modify exercises as necessary to ensure safety.

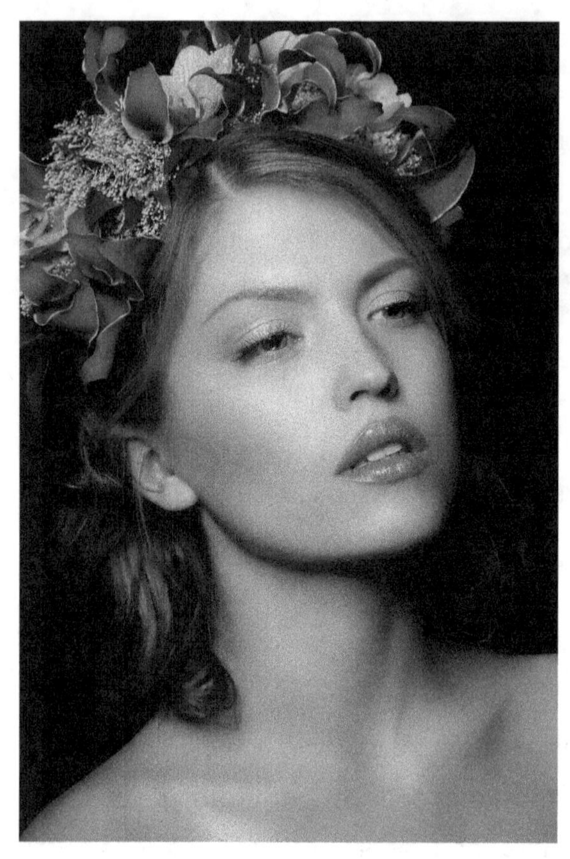

Chapter 5: Harnessing the Mind–Body Connection: Mindfulness and Meditation

Introduction to Mindfulness and Meditation:

In this chapter, we delve into the profound practice of mindfulness and meditation and explore their ability to strengthen the mind-body connection. Mindfulness is the practice of being fully present and aware of our thoughts, emotions, and physical sensations in the present moment, without judgment. Meditation, on the other hand, is a technique that involves training the mind to achieve a state of deep relaxation and emotional clarity.

The Science Behind Mindfulness and Meditation:

Scientific research has provided compelling evidence for the benefits of mindfulness and meditation on the mind and body. Studies have found that regular meditation can improve concentration, reduce stress, and increase resilience to emotional challenges. Neuroimaging studies have shown that meditation can lead to structural changes in the brain, strengthening connections between different regions and promoting emotional well-being. These practices have also been found to have positive effects on physical health, such as reducing blood pressure, improving sleep, and boosting the immune system.

Benefits of Mindfulness and Meditation:

The benefits of mindfulness and meditation are wide-ranging and have a profound impact on our overall well-being. Practicing mindfulness and meditation can help reduce stress and anxiety, promote a sense of calmand inner peace, improve focus and attention, enhance self-awareness, increase emotional intelligence, and foster a increased empathy and compassion for oneself and other people. These practices can also improve sleep quality, boost creativity, and enhance overall cognitive function.

Integrating Mindfulness and Meditation into Daily Life:

While mindfulness and meditation are often practiced during dedicated sessions, their true power lies in integrating them into our daily lives. By bringing a sense of mindfulness to everyday activities such as eating, walking, and interacting with others, we can cultivate a greater sense of presence and appreciation for the present moment. Simple mindfulness exercises, such as focusing on the breath or body sensations, can be practiced throughout the day to anchor our attention and reduce stress. Setting aside dedicated time for meditation can further deepen our practice and provide a space for introspection and relaxation.

Developing a Mindfulness and Meditation Practice:

To develop a mindfulness and meditation practice, it is important to start with small, manageable steps. Begin by carving out a few minutes each day for mindfulness meditation, finding a quiet space where you can sit comfortably and focus on your breath or a specific object of attention. As your practice becomes more established, gradually increase the duration and try different meditation techniques such as loving-kindness meditation or body scanmeditation. Additionally, exploring mindfulness in daily activities can be as simple as bringing attention to the sensations of eating or taking a walk in nature.

Overcoming Challenges and Cultivating Consistency:

Establishing a consistent mindfulness and meditation practice can sometimes be challenging. It is normal for the mind to wander or for obstacles to arise, such as restlessness or resistance. When these challenges arise, it is important to approach them with patience and self-compassion, gently guiding the attention back to the present moment. Joining a meditation group or seeking guidance from a qualified teacher can provide support and accountability. Additionally, integrating mindfulness reminders throughout the day, such as setting intention cues or using mobile apps, can help cultivate consistency in practice.

Mindfulness and meditation offer powerful tools for harnessing the mind-body connection and enhancing overall well-being. By cultivating present moment awareness and developing a deeper understanding of ourselves, we can experience reduced stress, increased focus, improved emotional balance, and a greater sense of overall fulfillment. Embracing these practices and integrating them into our daily lives allows us to tap into our innate inner wisdom and live more meaningful and purposeful lives.

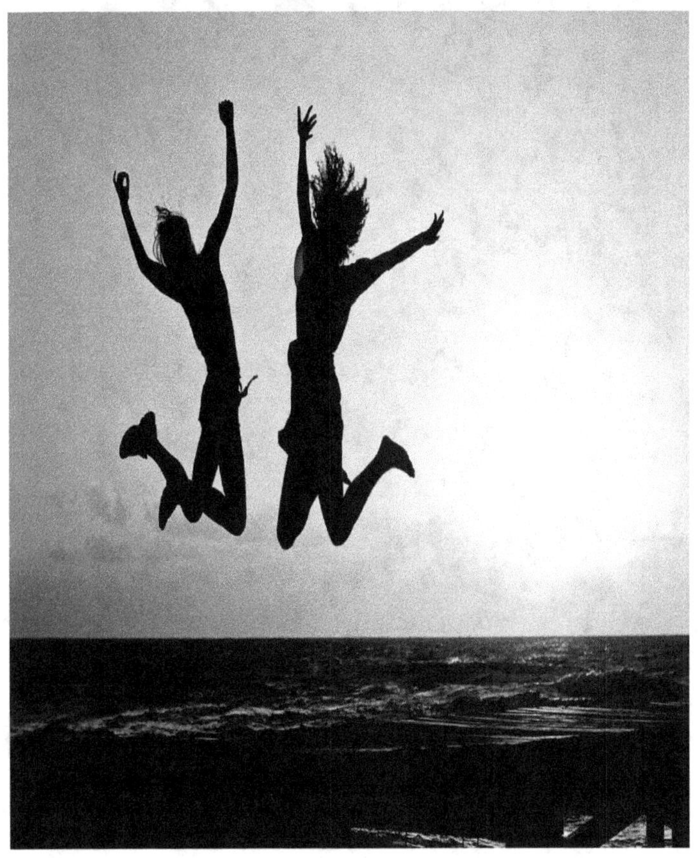

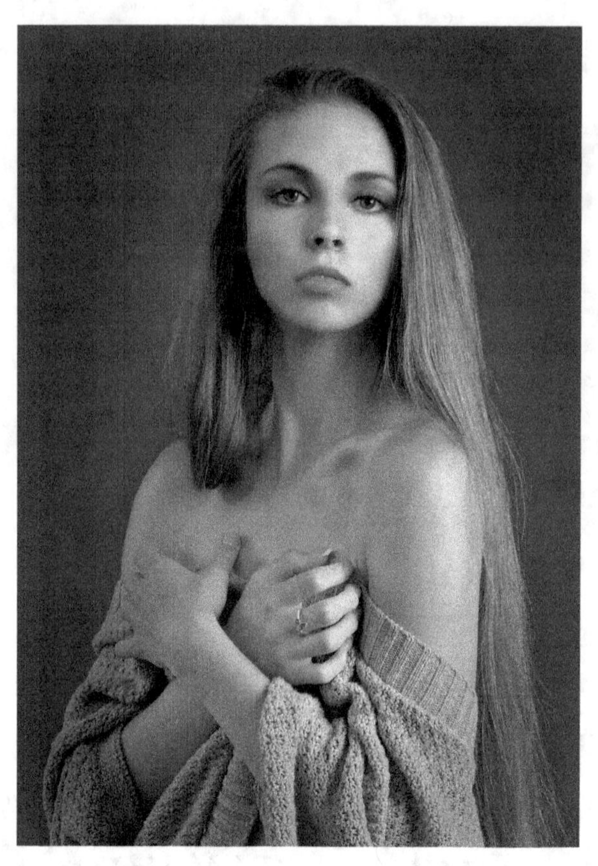

Chapter 6: Navigating Menopause and Hormonal Changes

Menopause is a natural process that occurs in women as they age, typically beginning in their late 40s or early 50s. It marks the end of a woman's reproductive years and is characterized by several hormonal changes within the body. These hormonal changes can cause a range of symptoms and may require some adjustments to maintain overall health and well-being.

During menopause, the production of hormones like estrogen and progesterone slows down and eventually ceases. This decrease in hormone levels can lead to a variety of physical and emotional symptoms. Hot flashes, night sweats, mood swings, weight gain, sleep disturbances, dry skin, and changes in sexual desire are some of the commonly reported symptoms. Each woman's experience with menopause is unique, and while some may experience these symptoms mildly, others may find them disruptive to their daily lives.

One of the most well-known symptoms of menopause is hot flashes. These sudden feelings of intense heat can occur multiple times a day and may be accompanied by sweating and a rapid heartbeat. Hot flashes can be uncomfortable and disruptive, but there are several strategies to manage them. Dressing in layers, avoiding triggers like spicy foods and caffeine, practicing deep breathing techniques, and keeping a fan nearby are some methods that may help alleviate hot flashes.

Chapter 7: Discovering the Benefits of Natural Supplements and Anti-aging Treatments

In the quest for eternal youth and vitality, many individuals are turning to natural supplements and anti-aging treatments. These alternative methods are gaining popularity due to their potential health benefits and minimal side effects compared to traditional pharmaceutical interventions. Chapter 7 delves into the world of natural supplements and anti-aging treatments, shedding light on their various benefits and how they can contribute to a healthier and more youthful life.

One of the primary benefits of natural supplements and anti-aging treatments is their ability to nourish and support the body from within. Unlike synthetic drugs that often target specific symptoms or conditions, natural supplements work holistically to enhance overall wellness. They are typically derived from natural sources such as herbs, vitamins, minerals, and other organic compounds.

These substances contain potent antioxidants and anti-inflammatory properties that can counteract the effects of aging and free radicals.

Anti-aging treatments, on the other hand, encompass a wide range of therapies and practices that aim to slow down or reverse the signs of aging. These treatments may include facial rejuvenation techniques, hormone replacement therapy, stem cell therapy, and various non-invasive procedures. By addressing the root causes of aging -- such as hormonal imbalances, cellular damage, and collagen loss -- these treatments can help improve skin elasticity, reduce wrinkles, boost energylevels, and promote overall vitality.

Another benefit of natural supplements and anti-aging treatments is their potential to strengthen the body's immune system. As we age, our immune system naturally weakens, making us more susceptible to illnesses and infections. By providing the body with essential nutrients and antioxidants, natural supplements can help support the immune system and enhance its ability to fight off pathogens. Anti-aging treatments, on the other hand, can stimulate the production of new immune cells and improve the body's defense mechanisms. Additionally, natural supplements and anti-aging treatments can contribute to improved cognitive function and mental clarity. Certain herbs and compounds found in natural supplements have been shown to enhance brain health, memory, and focus. Anti-aging treatments that target hormonal imbalances and cellular regeneration can also have a positive impact on cognitive function. By promoting healthy brain aging and reducing the risk of neurodegenerative diseases, these interventions can help maintain mental acuity and vitality.

Furthermore, natural supplements and anti-aging treatments can support cardiovascular health and prevent age-related diseases. Many natural supplements, such as Omega-3 fatty acids, CoQ10, and resveratrol, have been shown to promote heart health by reducing inflammation, improving blood flow, and lowering cholesterol levels. Anti-aging treatments thataddress the underlying causes of cardiovascular diseases, such as oxidative stress and arterial stiffness, can also have a positive impact on heart health. By including these interventions in a comprehensive anti-aging regimen, individuals can reduce their risk of heart disease and maintain a healthy cardiovascular system.

Lastly, natural supplements and anti-aging treatments can contribute to overall longevity and a higher quality of life. By addressing the various aspects of aging, such as physical health, mental well-being, and immune function, these interventions can help individuals live longer and healthier lives. Natural supplements and anti-aging treatments can also improve energy levels, promote better sleep, and enhance overall vitality, allowing individuals to enjoy an active and fulfilling lifestyle as they age.

In conclusion, chapter 7 explores the numerous benefits that natural supplements and anti-aging treatments can offer. From immune support and cognitive enhancement to cardiovascular health and longevity, these interventions have the potential to significantly improve overall well-being. By harnessing the power of nature and adopting a holistic approach to aging, individuals can embrace the benefits of natural supplements and anti-aging treatments to achieve a healthier, more youthful life.

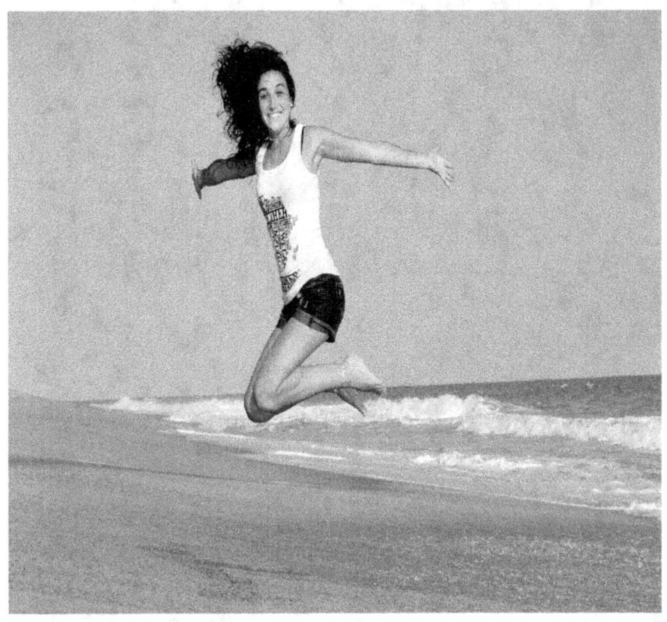

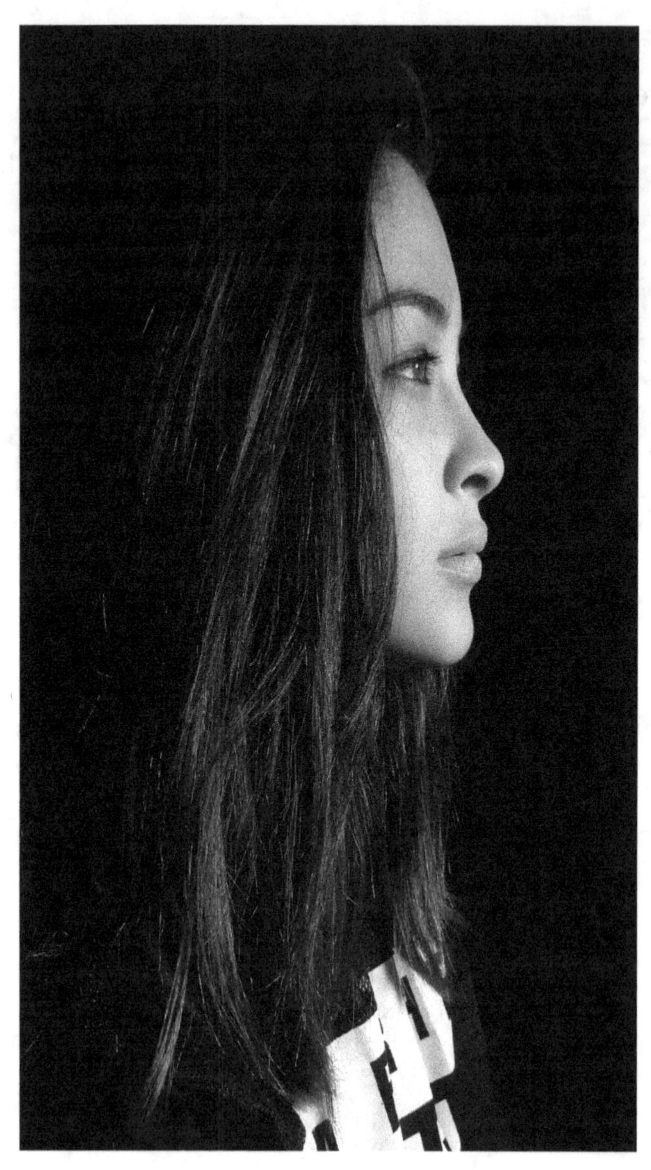

Chapter 8: Creating a Sustainable and Enjoyable Lifestyle: Finding Balance in Your Life

In the fast-paced and demanding world we live in, finding balance is often a challenge. Chapter 8 explores the importance of creating a sustainable and enjoyable lifestyle, and how finding balance can lead to a happier, healthier, and more fulfilling life.

One of the key aspects of creating a balanced lifestyle is prioritizing self-care. This means taking the time to nourish your body, mind, and soul. It's about ensuring that you are meeting your emotional, physical, and mental needs. Self-care can include activities such as exercising regularly, eating nutritious meals, getting enough sleep, practicing mindfulness or meditation, and engaging in hobbies or activities that bring you joy. By making self-care a priority, you can recharge and rejuvenate, which will ultimately enhance your overall well-being.

Another important element of a balanced lifestyle is managing stress effectively. In today's fast-paced world, stress is inevitable. However, it's how we handle and cope with stress that can make a big difference. Chapter 8 explores various stress management techniques that can help individuals maintain a sense of balance and calm. These techniques can include deep breathing exercises, practicing gratitude, engaging in regular physical activity, seeking social support, andsetting boundaries to prioritize self-care and personal time. By actively managing stress, individuals can prevent burnout and promote a more sustainable and enjoyable lifestyle.

Finding purpose and meaning in life is another crucial component of a balanced lifestyle. It's about aligning your actions and goals with your values and passions. Chapter 8 provides guidance on identifying your values, setting meaningful goals, and finding purpose in your daily activities. When you live a purpose-driven life, every action you take aligns with your core beliefs and brings you closer to a sense of fulfillment. This can create a profound sense of satisfaction and contentment, leading to a more balanced and enjoyable life.

Achieving work-life balance is also explored in chapter 8 as an essential aspect of a sustainable and enjoyable lifestyle. Balancing work demands with personal commitments can be challenging, but it is crucial for overall well-be

Chapter 9: Overcoming Challenges and Setting Realistic Goals

In life, challenges are inevitable. However, it is in our ability to overcome these challenges that we truly grow and achieve success. In Chapter 9, we will explore the importance of overcoming challenges and setting realistic goals to pave the way for accomplishing our dreams. This chapter aims to provide you with comprehensive strategies and insights to help you conquer obstacles, foster resilience, and set achievable goals that propel you towards a fulfilling life.

The Power of Overcoming Challenges

Acknowledging Challenges:

Challenges are a part of life that we all face at one point or another. They can be intimidating, overwhelming, and even discouraging. However, it is through facing and overcoming these challenges that we grow and develop as individuals.

The Power of Persistence:

Overcoming challenges requires persistence and the willingness to keep pushing forward, even when the going gets tough. It is about refusing to give up and finding the strength to continue moving towards your goals. It is through persistence that we are able to prove to ourselves and others that we have what it takes to overcome any obstacle in our path.

Building Resilience:

Overcoming challenges builds resilience, the ability to bounce back from setbacks and adapt to change. Resilience allows us to remain strong in the face of adversity and to keep moving forward, even when things don't go as planned. It is through these experiences that we become more resilient individuals, able to handle whatever life throws our way.

Unleashing Potential:

When we overcome challenges, we tap into a wellspring of untapped potential within ourselves. We discover what we are truly capable of and realize that we are capable of achieving anything we set our minds to. Overcoming challenges allows us to break free from the limitations we set for ourselves and to reach neheights of success and fulfillment.

Inspiring Others:

When we overcome challenges, we become an inspiration to others. Our stories of triumph serve as a reminder that anything is possible with determination and perseverance. By sharing our experiences, we can motivate and encourage others to overcome their own challenges and reach their full potential. We become a beacon of hope and a source of inspiration for those around us.

Personal Growth:

Ultimately, overcoming challenges is about personal growth. It's about growing into a more resilient, intelligent, and powerful person. Each challenge we face is an opportunity for growth and self-discovery. It is through these challenges that we learn valuable life lessons and become better equipped to handle future obstacles that come our way.

 The power of overcoming challenges should not be underestimated. It is through these experiences that we grow, build resilience, unleash our potential, inspire others, and achieve personal growth. So, embrace the challenges that come your way, for they hold the key to unlocking your true power and potential

Recognizing the significance of challenges as opportunities for growth and self-improvement.

Understanding that challenges act as catalysts for personal and professional development.

Challenges serve as catalysts for personal and professional development by pushing individuals outside their comfort zones and forcing them to acquire new skills and knowledge.

Overcoming challenges builds resilience and provides valuable learning experiences that can be applied to future endeavors.

Challenges enable self-reflection and self-improvement as individuals assess their strengths, weaknesses, and areas for growth.

When faced with challenges, individuals often discover hidden talents, creative problem-solving abilities, and increased confidence in their capabilities.

Professionally, challenges encourage individuals to think critically, innovate, and adapt to changing environments, fostering growth within organizations.

Successfully navigating challenges leads to personal satisfaction, increased self-esteem, and a greater sense of accomplishment.

Embracing challenges also widens one's perspective, fostering adaptability and open-mindedness, essential traits for personal and professional growth.

Challenges can foster collaboration and teamwork, as individuals come together to overcome obstacles and achieve common goals.

Ultimately, understanding that challenges act as catalysts for personal and professional development is crucial for individuals to embrace opportunities for growth, adapt to new situations, and realize their full potential.

Embracing Resilience:

Embracing resilience involves viewing challenges as opportunities for growth, developing coping mechanisms, and seeking support. Resilience fosters adaptability, enhances decision-making, and is valued in professional settings.

Cultivating emotional strength and adaptability to bounce back from setbacks.

Cultivating emotional strength involves building resilience and developing a positive mindset to effectively manage and regulate emotions during setbacks.

Adapting to setbacks requires a flexible and open-minded approach, allowing individuals to adjust their goals, strategies, and perspectives in response to adversity.

Embracing emotional strength and adaptability enables individuals to bounce back from setbacks, learn from their experiences, and emerge stronger and more capable.

It is essential to practice self-compassion and self-care, fostering emotional well-being and providing the foundation to navigate and overcome challenges.

Developing a growth mindset, embracing change, and seeking opportunities for personal and professional development contribute to building emotional strength and adaptability.

Emotionally strong and adaptable individuals possess the resilience to persevere through setbacks, overcome obstacles, and ultimately achieve their goals.

By cultivating emotional strength and adaptability, individuals are better equipped to navigate the inevitable ups and downs of life, fostering personal growth and success.

Developing a positive mindset that sees challenges as stepping stones to success.

Nurturing self-confidence and determination to navigate through difficult situations.

Learning from Setbacks:

Setbacks are inevitable in both personal and professional contexts. However, it is how we respond and learn from these setbacks that truly defines our growth and progress.

Learning from setbacks involves adopting a reflective mindset to evaluate the reasons behind the setback and identify areas for improvement. It requires acknowledging and accepting accountability for any mistakes or shortcomings.

By carefully analyzing setbacks, individuals gain valuable insights into what went wrong and acquire wisdom to avoid similar pitfalls in the future. This process enhances problem-solving skills and promotes continuous learning and growth.

Moreover, setbacks provide an opportunity for individuals to reassess their goals, priorities, and strategies. They can lead to a deeper understanding of individual strengths and weaknesses, enabling individuals to make adjustments and better align their actions with their aspirations.

Learning from setbacks also builds resilience and fosters adaptability. It empowers individuals to bounce back stronger, equipped with new strategies and renewed determination. It instills a sense of perseverance and a willingness to take calculated risks in the pursuit of success.

By embracing setbacks as valuable learning experiences, individuals develop a growth mindset and cultivate a more proactive approach to challenges. Their ability to learn from setbacks propels personal and professional development, leading to increased confidence and achievement of goals.

Extracting valuable lessons from failures and setbacks.

Failures and setbacks provide important opportunities for growth and learning.

By reflecting on failures, individuals can identify the factors that contributed to the setback and extract valuable lessons from the experience.

Understanding the root causes of failure helps individuals make necessary adjustments and improve their future performance.

Failures and setbacks can reveal hidden strengths and weaknesses, allowing individuals to focus on areas that require development.

Extracting lessons from failures promotes resilience, adaptability, and problem-solving skills.

It is important to approach failures with a growth mindset, embracing them as stepping stones towards success.

Valuable lessons learned from failures can lead to innovative approaches and more effective strategies.

Extracting lessons from setbacks builds self-awareness and fosters personal and professional growth.

Rather than dwelling on the failure itself, individuals can leverage the lessons learned to fuel future success.

Understanding that setbacks provide important insights for future growth and improvement.

Setbacks are not failures, but rather opportunities for growth and improvement. It is through setbacks that we gain valuable insights that can shape our paths to success.

Setbacks provide a unique perspective, highlighting areas that require further development and improvement. By reflecting on what went wrong, we can identify weaknesses, blind spots, and areas for growth.

These insights allow us to make necessary adjustments, adopt new approaches, and develop resilience. They empower us to learn from our mistakes and make informed decisions moving forward.

Moreover, setbacks provide a chance to reassess our goals, values, and priorities. They prompt us to refine our strategies, set new objectives, and align our actions with our long-term aspirations.

By understanding that setbacks are not roadblocks but rather learning opportunities, we can embrace them with a growth mindset. We learn to view setbacks as stepping stones towards future success, knowing that each setback brings us closer to our desired outcomes.

Ultimately, understanding that setbacks provide important insights for future growth and improvement enables us to navigate challenges with resilience, adaptability, and a commitment to continuous learning and advancement.

Embracing a growth mindset that focuses on learning rather than dwelling on failures.

A growth mindset is an empowering perspective that shifts the focus from dwelling on failures to embracing them as opportunities for learning and growth. By adopting a growth mindset, individuals develop a thirst for knowledge, resilience in the face of setbacks, and a belief in their ability to continually improve. Embracing this mindset allows individuals to view failures as stepping stones on the path to success, unlocking their full potential.

Building Support Networks:

Establishing a robust support system is crucial for both individual and occupational development. It involves surrounding oneself with individuals who provide guidance, encouragement, and assistance along the journey.

A support network offers various benefits. It provides a source of emotional support during challenging times, boosting resilience and mental well-being. It can also provide valuable insights and perspectives, helping individuals gain new knowledge and broaden their horizons.

To build a support network, it is important to nurture existing relationships and actively seek new connections. This can be done through networking events, professional organizations, or online platforms. Building genuine, mutually beneficial relationships fosters a sense of community and creates opportunities for collaboration and mentorship.

Additionally, offering support to others within one's network creates a reciprocal environment of trust and camaraderie. This helps foster a sense of belonging and provides a supportive ecosystem where individuals can thrive.

Building a support network requires active effort and commitment. Regular communication, mutual respect, and a willingness to contribute are vital for nurturing and maintaining these vital connections.

Ultimately, building a strong support network equips individuals with the resources and encouragement needed to navigate challenges and achieve personal and professional success

Recognizing the importance of having a strong support system.

Having a strong support system is crucial for personal growth and well-being. It offers motivation, emotional support, and a feeling of community. It helps navigate challenges and celebrates accomplishments. Recognizing the importance of a strong support system is essential for building resilience and fostering meaningful connections.

Building a network of mentors, peers, and friends who can provide guidance, encouragement, and advice during challenging times.

Building a network of mentors, peers, and friends is crucial for navigating the ups and downs of life. Surrounding yourself with individuals who can offer guidance, encouragement, and advice during challenging times can be immensely valuable. These connections can provide a support system that offers different perspectives, experiences, and expertise. By actively seeking out and nurturing relationships with individuals who inspire and challenge you, you create a network that can help you overcome obstacles, provide reassurance, and offer a sounding board when needed. It is through these meaningful connections that personal growth and resilience thrive.

Seeking professional assistance, if needed, to tackle specific challenges.

Seeking professional assistance when facing specific challenges is a wise decision. Sometimes, despite our best efforts, certain problems require expertise beyond our own capabilities. Professional assistance can provide specialized knowledge, skills, and guidance tailored to tackle those particular obstacles. Whether it's seeking therapy, consulting an expert, or joining support groups, these resources can equip us with tools and strategies to overcome our challenges. Recognizing the value of professional help demonstrates strength and a commitment to personal growth. So, don't hesitate to reach out when necessary – it's a step toward finding effective solutions and ultimately improving our well-being.

Setting Realistic Goals

Setting realistic goals is essential for success. It is important to consider your abilities, resources, and time constraints when determining what goals you can realistically achieve. Setting unrealistic goals can lead to disappointment and frustration, while setting realistic goals allows you to stay motivated and gives you a clear path towards accomplishment.

Defining Success:

Defining success is a personal and subjective matter. It goes beyond financial achievements or societal recognition. Success can be defined as the fulfillment of personal goals, finding joy and satisfaction in one's endeavors, maintaining healthy relationships, and striving for personal growth and happiness. Ultimately, success is about living a meaningful and fulfilling life in alignment with your values and purpose.

Understanding that success is personal and varies from individual to individual.

I hope this note finds you well. I wanted to take a moment to remind you of something very important - success is personal and unique to each individual. In today's society, we often find ourselves comparing our achievements to others, which can be disheartening. However, it is crucial to remember that success is not a one-size-fits-all concept. Each person has their own goals, aspirations, and definitions of what success means to them.

While one person may consider financial stability as the epitome of success, another might prioritize personal relationships or pursuing their passions.Respecting and recognizing these differences is crucial.

Instead of measuring your success against others', focus on your own journey. Celebrate the milestones you have achieved, no matter how big or small they may seem. Remember, success is subjective, and what matters most is whether you feel fulfilled and content with your own accomplishments.

Keep striving towards your goals, setting your own standards, and trusting that your version of success is valid. Embrace the uniqueness of your journey, as it is what makes you who you are.

Clarifying your own definition of success based on your values, passions, and aspirations.

Clarifying your own definition of success involves understanding your values, passions, and aspirations. It requires identifying what truly matters to you and what brings you fulfillment. Success is not solely measured by external achievements or societal standards, but by personal growth and contentment. By aligning your actions with your values, pursuing your passions, and working towards your aspirations, you can define your own version of success that brings you joy and satisfaction. Success becomes a reflection of living a meaningful and purposeful life, while staying true to yourself

Importance of Realistic Goals:

Setting realistic goals is crucial for success. They allow us to focus our efforts, stay motivated, and make progress towards our desires. Realistic goals provide a clear path to follow, ensuring we don't get overwhelmed or discouraged. They help us prioritize and tackle challenges more effectively. By setting achievable targets, we build our confidence and self-belief, which propels us further. Realistic goals also give us a sense of direction and purpose, keeping us on track and guiding our decision-making. Ultimately, they lead us to success by keeping us grounded, focused, and motivated while we work towards our aspirations.

Recognizing the significance of setting goals that are attainable and feasible within your current circumstances.

Recognizing the significance of setting attainable and feasible goals within our current circumstances is key to success. While it's important to dream big, setting goals that align with our realities is vital for progress. Attainable goals allow us to thrive in the present, making the most of our resources and abilities. They prevent us from feeling overwhelmed or discouraged, maintaining our motivation along the way. Feasible goals ensure practicality, considering our current circumstances, such as time, finances, and commitments. By setting attainable and feasible goals, we create a roadmap that is realistic and sustainable, increasing our chances of success and fulfillment. Remember, Recall that success involves both enjoying the journey and arriving at the objective.

Avoiding the trap of setting overly ambitious goals that can lead to discouragement and burnout.

When setting goals, it's important to be realistic and avoid setting overly ambitious goals that are too difficult or unrealistic to achieve.

By setting goals that are too ambitious, you may set yourself up for failure, which can lead to discouragement and eventually burnout.

- It's important to set goals that are attainable and aligned with your abilities, resources, and time constraints.

Divide more ambitious objectives into more doable tasks or benchmarks. This helps to make progress more tangible and keeps you motivated along the way.

Remember Recall that achievement is a process rather than a final goal.

 success is a journey, not a destination. Celebrate small victories and acknowledge the progress you make towards your goals.

Regularly review and reassess your goals. If you find that a goal is too ambitious or no longer aligns with your needs or priorities, it's okay to adjust or change it.

Lastly, prioritize self-care and wellbeing. Avoid overworking or exerting yourself to the point of burnout. Listen to your body and mind, and make sure to take breaks, rest, and relax when needed.

SMART Goal Setting:

SMART goal setting is a powerful technique that helps individuals and teams plan for success. Specific, Measurable, Achievable, Relevant, and Time-bound is what the acronym SMART stands for. This method provides a structured and systematic approach to goal setting, ensuring that objectives are clear, well-defined, and realistic.

Specificity is the first aspect of SMART goal setting. By clearly defining what you want to achieve, you give yourself a clear target to aim for. Rather to stating general objectives such as "I want to lose weight," a more targeted objective may be "I want to lose 10 pounds in the next 3 months." This lucidity enables you to focus your efforts and determine the necessary steps to reach your goal.

The second component of SMART goal setting is measurability. By establishing tangible metrics to assess your progress, you can track your journey towards accomplishing your goal. In our previous example, the measurable aspect would be the 10 pounds you want to lose. Measuring your progress along the way keeps you motivated and provides a sense of accomplishment.

Achievability is the third component of SMART goal setting. It's important to set goals that are challenging but still within reach. If a goal seems too difficult or impossible, it can be demotivating. However, if your goals are too simple, you might not be motivated to realize your full potential.By ensuring your goals are achievable, you set yourself up for success and maintain a sense of motivation and determination.

The fourth component of SMART goal setting is relevance. It's crucial to set goals that align with your overarching objectives and values. Your goals should be meaningful to you and contribute to your personal or professional growth. When your goals are relevant, you are more likely to stay committed and focused on achieving them.

Finally, time-bound refers to setting a deadline for achieving your goal. By establishing a specific timeframe, you create a sense of urgency and keep yourself accountable. The deadline provides a sense of structure and helps you prioritize your actions to stay on track.

In summary, SMART goal setting is an effective approach to achieving success. By making your goals Specific, Measurable, Achievable, Relevant, and Time-bound, you give yourself the best chance of reaching your desired outcomes. So, whether you're aiming for personal improvement, career advancement, or team performance, utilizing the SMART goal setting technique can greatly enhance your chances of success.

Introducing the SMART (Specific, Measurable, Achievable, Relevant, Time-bound) framework for setting goals.

Breaking down big goals into smaller, manageable steps.

Defining clear metrics to measure progress and success.

Aligning Goals with Values:

I trust this note finds you well. I wanted to share a brief but captivating perspective on the importance of aligning our goals with our values.

Aligning our goals with our values is the key to unlocking a life of true fulfillment and purpose. When our goals are in harmony with our values, it ignites a powerful synergy that propels us towards success fueled by authenticity.

By consciously aligning our goals with our values, we ensure that our actions are a true reflection of who we are and what we believe in. This alignment brings clarity, meaning, and a profound sense of fulfillment to our daily pursuits.

When we let our values guide our goals, we remain grounded in our authentic selves. We make choices that resonate with our core beliefs and aspirations, fostering a deep sense of alignment and satisfaction.

On the other hand, pursuing goals that do not align with our values can leave us feeling unsatisfied and disconnected from our true purpose. Therefore, it is essential to reflect on what truly matters to us and let these values shape our goal-setting process.

Aspire to live a life where your goals and values are in harmony. Embrace the journey of discovering what truly matters to you, and allow these values to guide and inspire your every goal and action.

Ensuring that your goals align with your core values and principles.

Prioritizing goals that resonate deeply with your passions and beliefs, increasing motivation and fulfillment.

Strategies for Overcoming Challenges and Achieving Realistic Goals

Overcoming challenges and achieving realistic goals can often feel like an uphill battle. However, with the right strategies, you can navigate obstacles and make your goals a reality. Here are some effective approaches to help you on your journey:

1. Break it down: Large goals can be overwhelming. Break them down into smaller, manageable tasks. This will make your goals feel more achievable and help you stay motivated along the way.

2. Prioritize and focus: Identify the most important tasks that will directly contribute to your goal. Prioritize these tasks and give them your full attention. By focusing on what truly matters, you can make significant progress and stay on track.

3. Adapt and learn: Challenges are inevitable, but they also provide an opportunity for growth. Embrace them as learning experiences and adapt your approach when necessary. Be open to new ideas and perspectives that can help you overcome obstacles.

4. Seek support: Don't be afraid to ask for help. Embrace a network of mentors, family members, or friends who are willing to assist and guide you Collaborating with others can bring fresh insights and help you overcome challenges more effectively.

5. Stay positive and resilient: Maintaining a positive mindset is crucial. Believing in yourself and your ability to overcome challenges will keep you motivatedand resilient. Celebrate small victories along the way and stay focused on the progress you are making, even in the face of setbacks.

6. Plan and track progress: Create a detailed plan outlining the steps you need to take to achieve your goals. Break it down into specific timelines and milestones. Regularly track your progress to stay accountable and make adjustments as necessary.

7. Take care of yourself: Self-care is essential for maintaining the energy and focus needed to overcome challenges and achieve goals. Prioritize your physical and mental well-being by getting enough rest, exercising, eating nutritious foods, and managing stress.

8. Stay organized and disciplined: Develop good organizational habits to maximize productivity. Use tools such as calendars, to-do lists, and productivity apps to stay organized and disciplined. Establish routines that support your goal achievement journey.

Remember that challenges are a natural part of the journey towards achieving realistic goals. By implementing these strategies, you can overcome obstacles with resilience and determination. Stay focused, adapt when needed, and celebrate your progress along the way. You've got this!

Developing an Action Plan:

Developing an action plan is the key to turning dreams into achievable realities. It provides a roadmap to guide your efforts and keep you on track. Here's how you can create an effective action plan:

1. Define your goal: Clearly articulate what you want to achieve. A specific and measurable goal will help you stay focused and track progress.

2. Break it down: Divide your goal into smaller, manageable tasks. This makes it less overwhelming and easier to tackle one step at a time.

3. Set deadlines: Establish realistic timelines for each task. Deadlines create a sense of urgency and help you stay committed to your plan.

4. Prioritize: Identify the most important tasks that will have the greatest impact on reaching your goal. Focus on these first to maximize your efforts.

5. Take action: Start working on your tasks. Procrastination only delays progress. Start small and gain momentum from there.

6. Track progress: Regularly review and measure your progress. This allows you to assess what's working and make any necessary adjustments to your plan.

7. Stay motivated: Find ways to stay motivated and inspired throughout the process. Celebrate small wins and remind yourself of the benefits of achieving your goal.

8. Seek support: Don't hesitate to ask forhelp or guidance along the way. Surrounding yourself with a supportive network or seeking expert advice can provide valuable insights and encouragement.

Remember, developing an action plan is the catalyst for turning your aspirations into reality. With careful planning, prioritization, and consistent action, you can make significant progress towards your goal. Stay focused, adapt as needed, and celebrate each milestone on your journey to success.

- Creating a structured and detailed plan of action to achieve your goals.

Breaking down big goals into smaller, actionable tasks.

Setting deadlines for each task to create a sense of urgency and accountability.

Adopting a Growth Mindset:

Unlock your potential: Embrace a growth mindset and watch yourself soar beyond imagined limits.

- Embracing the belief that intelligence and abilities can be developed with effort and learning.

- Viewing challenges as opportunities for personal growth and skill development.

- Being open to feedback and continuously seeking opportunities to learn and improve.

Cultivating Discipline and Persistence:

- Cultivating self-discipline to stay focused and committed to your goals.

- Developing habits and routines that align with your objectives.

- Persisting in the face of adversity, setbacks, and obstacles.

Seeking Continuous Learning:

- Prioritizing personal and professional growth through continuous learning.

- Engaging in self-improvement activities such as reading, attending workshops, or acquiring new skills.

- Seeking out mentors and experts who can provide guidance and insights.

Celebrating Milestones and Seeking Support:

- Celebrating small victories and milestones along the way to stay motivated.

- Recognizing and appreciating progress, no matter how small.

- Seeking support from your support network during challenging times, both for emotionaland practical assistance.

Chapter 9 emphasizes the importance of overcoming challenges and setting realistic goals on the path to success. By acknowledging challenges, nurturing resilience, and learning from setbacks, you can develop the strength and mindset necessary to overcome any obstacle. Setting realistic goals aligned with your values, utilizing the SMART framework, and adopting a growth mindset will help you stay focused and motivated in pursuing your aspirations. Additionally, implementing strategies such as developing an action plan, cultivating discipline and persistence, seeking continuous learning, and seeking support from your network will provide the necessary tools for overcoming challenges and achieving your goals. Remember, both challenges and goals are opportunities for personal growth and fulfillment. With the right mindset and strategies, you can conquer any obstacle and create a life of success, happiness, and contentment.

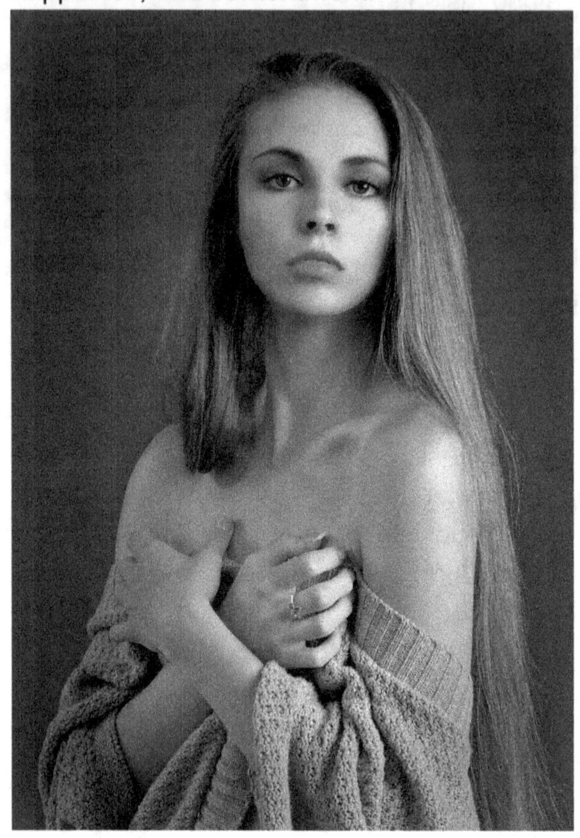

Chapter 10: Embracing Your Fit and and Fabulous Future: Celebrating Your Achievements

Congratulations! You have come a long way on your journey of personal growth and transformation. In this final chapter, we invite you to reflect on your achievements and embrace the limitless possibilities that lie ahead.

As you look back on your progress, take a moment to truly celebrate your achievements. Each milestone reached, every goal accomplished, and every challenge overcome has shaped you into the empowered individual you are today. Recognize the strength, resilience, and determination that brought you this far.

Embracing your fit and fabulous future begins with acknowledging and honoring all that you have accomplished. It's a time to revel in your successes and bask in the glow of your victories, big and small. Allow yourself to feel proud of the progress you have made and the person you have become.

But celebration doesn't just stop at patting yourself on the back. It's also about looking forward and harnessing the momentum of your achievements to propel yourself towards an even more extraordinary future. This is your opportunity to dream bigger, set new goals, and design the life you've always envisioned.

Now that you have cultivated a growth mindset, you understand that there are no limits to what you can achieve. Yourachievements are not endpoints but stepping stones to greater heights. Use this chapter to reflect on the lessons learned along the way and to chart a course for your future endeavors.

It's crucial to maintain a sense of gratitude throughout this process. Express appreciation for the support of loved ones, mentors, and allies who have stood by your side. Remember that your success is not solely an individual accomplishment but a result of collective effort and collaboration.

As you celebrate your achievements and step into your fit and fabulous future, continue to challenge yourself. Seek out new opportunities to learn, grow, and evolve. Embrace discomfort and push beyond your comfort zone, knowing that great rewards often come from taking courageous leaps.

In this chapter, you will find exercises and prompts to help you reflect on your accomplishments, set new goals, and create an actionable plan for the future. Remember, this is not the end of your journey but a launching pad for even greater achievements.

Embrace your fit and fabulous future with enthusiasm and confidence. Celebrate your achievements and let them fuel your pursuit of a life filled with purpose, fulfillment, and endless possibilities. Your future is yours to create, and with a growth mindset, the sky is truly the limit.

Cheers to your extraordinary journey and the limitless potential that lies ahead!

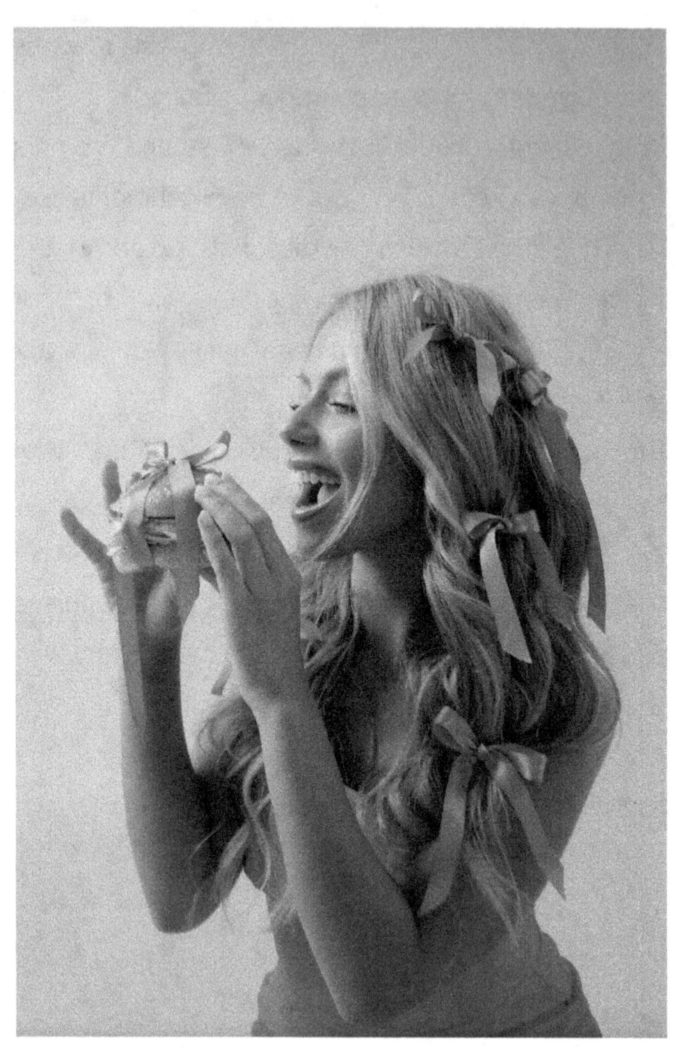

Conclusion: Your Personal Roadmap to Looking 20 Again

"Your Personal Roadmap to Looking 20" is an indispensable guide that will transform your appearance and boost your confidence. It offers you a comprehensive roadmap to uncovering your true beauty and unlocking your greatest potential. By diving into this treasure trove of skincare tips, fashion advice, and lifestyle techniques, you are embarking on a journey that will revolutionize your self-image and leave you radiating with youthful brilliance.

But the journey doesn't end here. As you continue this remarkable transformation, you will discover that the pages of this book are just the beginning of a lifelong quest for beauty and self-discovery. Armed with the knowledge and tools provided, you will unlock endless possibilities and continue to harness the power of your unique beauty.

So why stop now? By delving deeper into "Your Personal Roadmap to Looking 20," you will gain an unwavering confidence and a timeless sense of style. You will learn how to conquer the aging process with grace and elegance, and you will confidently navigate the world as a beacon of beauty-inspiring others to do the same.

Remember, beauty is not just skin deep. It resonates from within, and "Your Personal Roadmap to Looking 20" will guide you towards nurturing that inner radiance. With everyturn of the page, you will uncover new ways to enhance your beauty, boost your self-esteem, and express your true essence.

Furthermore, "Your Personal Roadmap to Looking 20" will continue to be your trusted companion in the ever-evolving world of beauty and fashion. As trends come and go, this book remains a timeless resource, equipping you with the knowledge to adapt and stay ahead of the game. Whether it's the latest skincare breakthrough or an innovative fashion statement, you can trust that this book will keep you at the forefront of the industry.

Investing in "Your Personal Roadmap to Looking 20" is an investment in yourself. It is a commitment to becoming the best version of yourself and embracing your unique beauty. So don't hesitate to continue down this transformative path. Keep indulging in the wisdom, inspiration, and practical advice found within these pages, and watch as your beauty radiates from the inside out.

Get ready to embark on a journey that will not only change the way you look but also how you feel. With "Your Personal Roadmap to Looking 20," the possibilities are endless, and your beauty knows no bounds. So don't wait any longer; make the decision to prioritize yourself and continue investing in this invaluable resource. Youdeserve to look and feel your absolute best, and "Your Personal Roadmap to Looking 20" will be your steadfast guide every step of the way. Embrace this opportunity to transform your appearance, enhance your self-confidence, and unlock the true beauty that lies within you. The journey begins now.

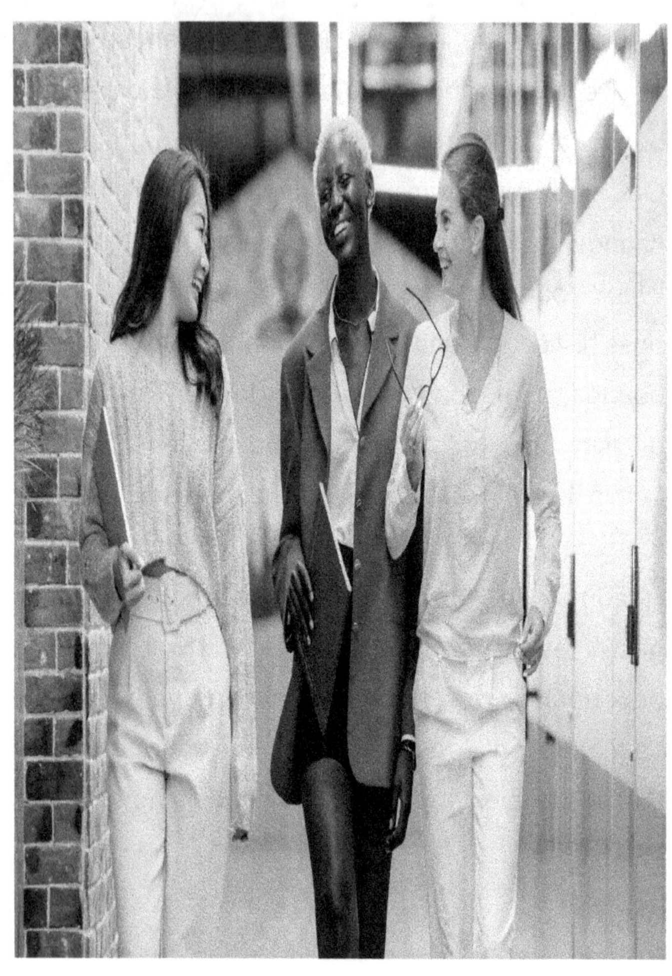

www.ingramcontent.com/pod-product-compliance
Lightning Source LLC
Chambersburg PA
CBHW061002260726
48661CB00005B/2001